Coming to America by Air

and

How American Food
and a Western Lifestyle Led Me
to Gain Over 100 Pounds

by

Betty Beatrice Akinyi Odak

INTRODUCTION:

On April 14, 2011, a nurse from my doctor's office called and said *"Betty, it is official, you are diabetic. You need to come to the office and pick up diabetic medication and a kit for checking your blood sugar"*. We made the necessary arrangements and then the nurse hung up the phone.

My life had changed. I was sitting down when she called. I do not recall how long I sat on that chair. I knew what the disease could do to a person. I remembered family members from my ex-husband's side that had died of diabetes. I pictured myself without a leg or an eye, consequences of this life threatening disease. I could feel my anxiety, depression and adrenalin climbing higher as my dread grew even deeper. I knew that I would not wait to have that happen to me, especially if there was something I could do to reverse the situation.

I walked to the pharmacy and picked up the medications. I did not know it then but I had already taken the first step to controlling the disease. It would not be easy. I had high blood pressure, high cholester ol and I was taking more than 10 pills every day. I was determined to make changes to my health no matter the cost. At that moment, I knew I needed to change my life. I knew that I needed to lose weight or lose my life.

I came to the U.S. from Nairobi, Kenya on Labor Day, September 3, 1995 as an undergraduate student. My weight was one hundred and fifty (150) pounds.

During my college years at Biola University in La Mirada, I gained about seventy pounds (70 lbs.) in four years-about 17.5 pounds every month.

It wasn't hard to put on the weight in the U.S. In Kenya, pizza is quite expensive but it was readily available and very cheap around my college campus. In fact, it wouldn't be hard to find the same situation around any American college campus. Cheap fast food, heavy with carbohydrates, are a significant part of many young people's diets. With limited access to a kitchen and limited time for buying and preparing my own foods, I made the same choices other students made when it came to meals.

The cheap foods in Kenya were fruits and vegetables. Hamburgers and fries were expensive in my native country. Although fruits and vegetables are cheap here, too, I couldn't resist treating myself to what would have been a Kenyan luxury item. Everyone back home would have been amazed at the cost I paid for a hamburger meal and even more astonished at the number of fast food choices that were available to me every day.

Most Kenyans walk to places. Things are changing now with people owning their own cars and/or using public transportation. However, in the rural areas, walking is still a means of transportation.

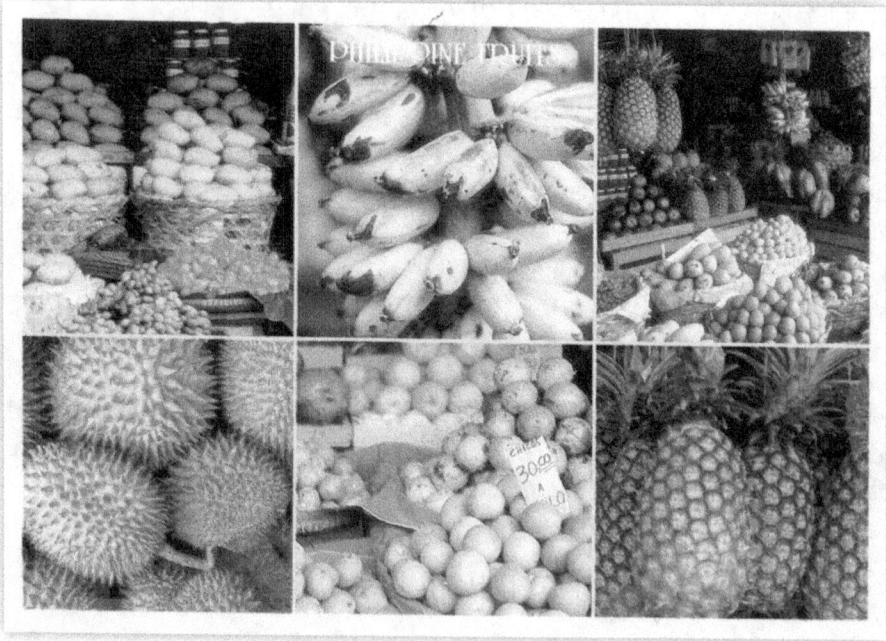

Low carbohydrate dieting has become stylish in recent years especially with the publication of the Atkins diet. Losing weight is a goal for so many people and everybody is looking for the quick and easy way to lose weight. Some people do not need to lose weight at all but still stressed and obsessed over a couple of pounds. Others need to lose for medical reasons and may have one hundred pounds or more that they want to shed.

At Biola University, I worked at the student cafeteria, which provided me with free food, many choices, and my weight began to increase daily.

I gained more weight after leaving college than at any other time in my entire life. By 2009, I weighed two hundred and ninety (290) pounds but I had already begun to pay the price for living in the land of abundance. I was taking three kinds of pills for various medical conditions. I felt awkward looking at myself in the mirror. I was constantly tired and any small walk up the stairs was like climbing Mount Kilimanjaro.

By this time, I had stopped any small exercise I was doing. I would eat convenient foods; order pizza, buy a dollar hamburgers and sodas, bread and peanut butter.

I was very unhappy that I had lived in the U.S. for over fifteen years and was still struggling with legal papers.

I was unhappy because I lost my only job at the time. I was unhappy because of one of my daughter's and sister's negative behaviors. At some point, I thought no American man would be interested in me because of my weight. I met one person through eHarmony – online dating, but when I told him my weight, he backed off. This made me depressed and felt people, especially the opposite sex were only interested in my physical appearance, but not my intellect and charm.

I was in trouble, physically and emotionally and there did not seem to be a solution.

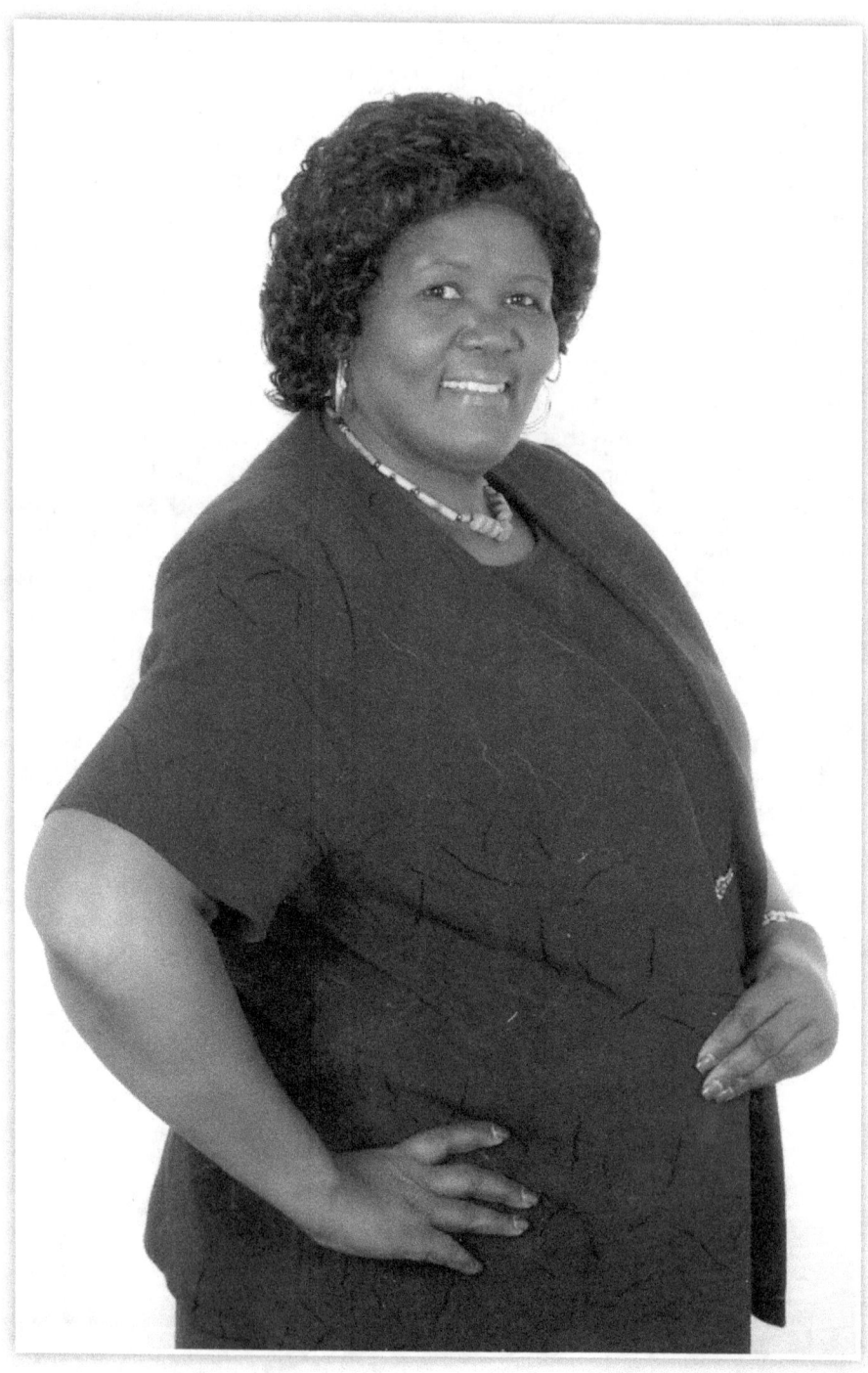

CHAPTER I
Early Life and Growing up in Kenya

I am the first born of twelve children. I grew up in a polygamous home. My father had two wives. I grew up in a small village called Wire Kabeka, in Oyugis division. Wire Kabeka was named after the first missionaries in that town. Wire is a small village with about two hundred people who know each other. It is located in the Southern part of Nyanza Province and three h u n d r e d m i l e s f r o m Nairobi, the capital city of Kenya. Nearby cities are Kisii and Homa-Bay. Most people who live in Wire village grow potatoes, maize, and millet as their cash crops. The majority of people grow their own vegetables, like collard greens, cabbages, tomatoes, onions, oranges, guavas, papayas, oranges, bananas, and avocados.

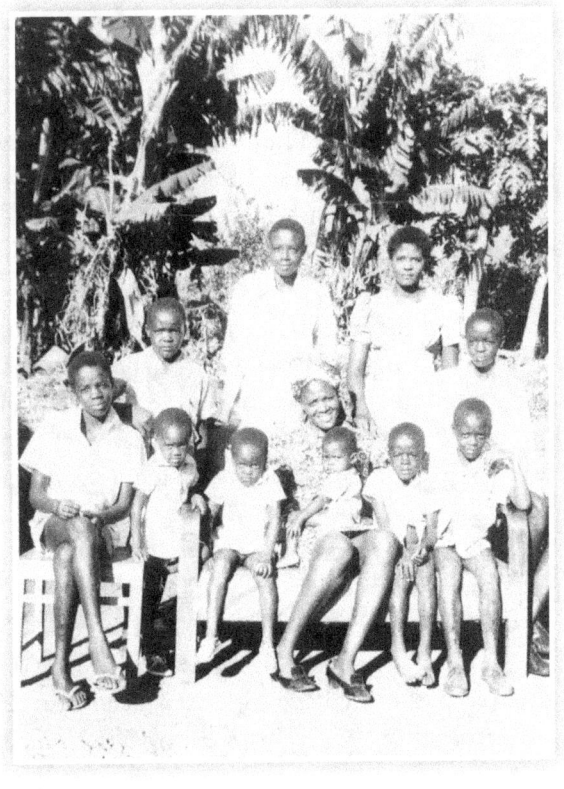

Food was scarce at home. I remember my mother would buy one big tilapia fish (ngege) and divide it amongst all of us. My youngest sister liked the head and we complained that she got more fish than the rest of us. The other food that was common was collard greens and cooked grinded maize. Breakfast was sweet potatoes or cooked bananas and black tea. Sometimes, if my mother could afford it, we had tea with milk. Porridge was popular. Bread was a luxury.

We ate bread probably once a week when there was a guest at home. My mother did not want to show that we could not afford certain necessities. We ate breakfast before going to school and would come back for lunch if there were left over's.

In the evening we always ate collard greens and cooked grinded maize (sukuma wiki and ugali). There was no television so we all went to bed by 8:00 pm. Sometimes we would listen to the radio until 9:00 pm.

My mother had two best friends who helped in time of need. Mr. and Mrs. Obura always came to our rescue. Mrs. Omondi who worked with East African Industries brought us blue band, washing detergent and tooth pastes. Those were happy days!

However, all girls attaining the age of ten were expected to sleep at their grand- mothers. At age ten, I also joined the other girls to sleep at my grandmother's house. We all slept on one mat with one blanket. I always slept in the middle because I could be assured of being warm at night. Upon waking up, I had mat marks all over my body. There was no bed or mattress. I would wake up with marks on my body from the sleeping mat and the other children would tease me about it. They knew I slept on a mat not a mattress. This kind of bullying made me sad and angry, but I was in good health during my childhood.

All of us girls slept at my grandmother's house. This was a way of protecting us from bad influences. It was also a time for my grandmother to tell us stories and moral lessons. My grandmother had trouble sleeping and she would tell many stories each night. We would fall asleep before the third story. She got mad if we fell asleep before she finished all her stories.

My grandmother cooked the best meals. I loved her food. She used clay pots and firewood. She cooked the best meat ever! My grandmother was very healthy because of the food she ate. She never ate eggs, milk, chicken or raw meat. She lived to be 103 years old and still had her own teeth. I must have inherited her genes. People say I have beautiful teeth and my grandmother's teeth were beautiful too.

It was effortless to stay healthy. Everything we did was by hand. No extra effort was made to do exercise. We walked to school, church, market, river, and the mountain and at the end of the day; we were all tired, ate and went to sleep.

The means of transportation for most people was on foot, unless it was a long journey of over fifty miles. We would even come home for lunch and ran back to school. There were pebbles and stones in the road but we ran bare footed.

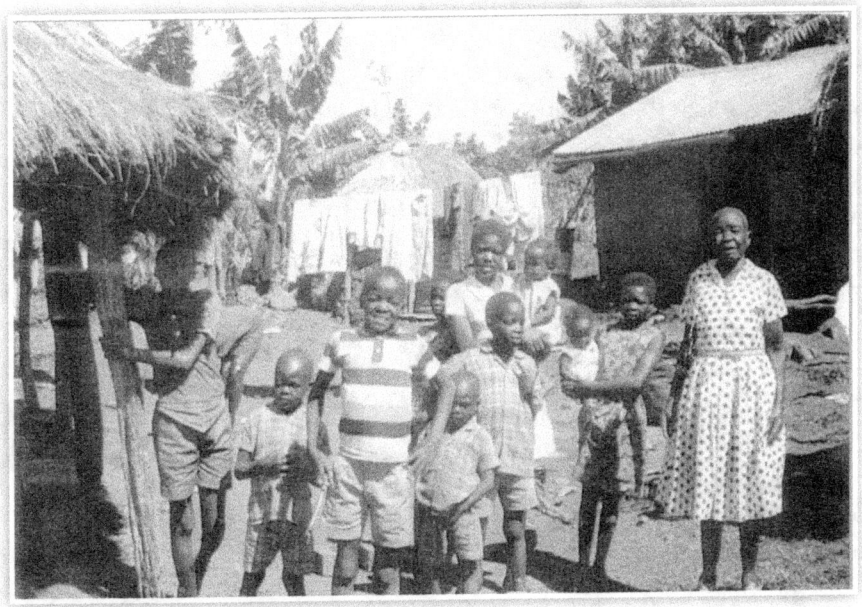

I got my first pair or rubber shoes when I was in sixth grade. Gee was I excited. Unfortunately, I would not even wear those shoes because I did not want them to get dirty. I waited too long because my feet became too big for the shoes. Well, I could not give them to my brother because they were women's shoes. My father bought me another pair of shoes a year later. I could only wear these shoes when going to church or some important places like Sports day or the Independence Day celebration, Jamhuri Day.

Walking to school was fun even during the rainy seasons. My two best friends Alice, Akoth, and I were always together. We were known as the triple A's – Akinyi, Alice, Akoth. Danish was also one of my best friends. He came from a rich family and had shoes most of the time. Sometimes I would ask him to loan me his shoes. Danish and I formed a very close childhood relationship. Danish was a pastor's son. In their house was electricity, which made us feel they were very rich. He was kind and protected me many times when others tried to beat me up. We are still friends even today. He is now married with children.

The Triple A group was dismantled after primary school. We all went to different secondary schools, but continued our friendship through written correspondence. Of course we saw each other during school holidays.

Most Kenyan boarding schools are segregated by sexes. I went to Dudi Girls High School. This was a community (harambee) based school. It was a very poor high school with no running water or electricity. We had to go draw water from a nearby river and carry it on our heads before going to classes. The river was more than ten miles away from the school. I hated this school. However, I was involved in sports like volley ball, netball and track and field.

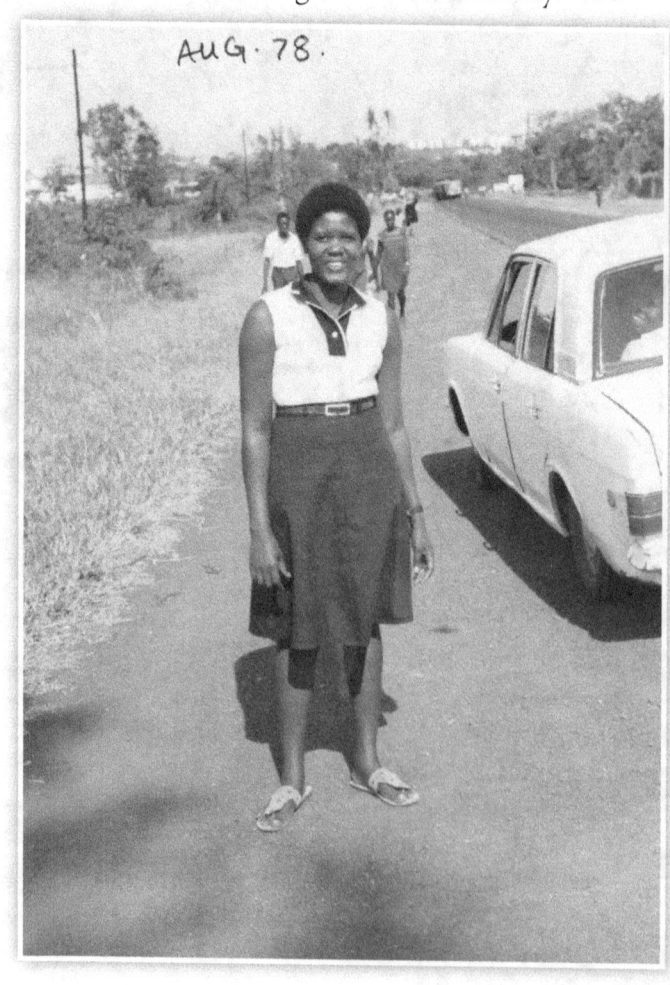

The food came from the school garden. All these activities and fresh food made my body strong and healthy. Boarding school food was horrible. The school had rules that no one can bring food from outside or buy from a near- by grocery store. The school prefect forced us to eat cafeteria food. But food was measured and served to each student. We were given one scoop of baked beans, some maize and over- cooked cabbage.

Desert was either a piece of banana or orange. I lost a lot of weight during that time. I was very sick and had to go home for treatment.

After two semesters, I joined Ogande Girls High School in Homa-Bay dis- trict. This was a government school and very prestigious. I liked it a lot. It had running water and a generator for electricity. I had always been scared of darkness even though back at home, we never had electricity at the time. I was very outgoing and charming. I became class prefect in the first form (first year). This excluded me from doing other chores like cleaning the stinking toilets, cleaning the dormitories, or digging. I was elected school prefect on my second year in school and all the years thereafter until I graduated from high school. I thoroughly enjoyed my secondary school years. I was involved in different kinds of sports — like volley ball which I played up to national level, netball and tennis. I stayed fit doing all these exercises. Weight gain was not an issue. There was always fresh food available. Fruits like bananas, oranges, mangos, guavas, avocados and papayas were homegrown.

I was a very happy child and had many friends. My father loved me though he died unexpectedly when I was a teenager. I was unhappy many times because my mother expected me to cook for everybody. We used firewood, which at times was very difficult to start, especially if the firewood was not dry enough, or it damp because of the rain. I loved going to school because at home I was always responsible for my siblings being I was the first-born.

CHAPTER 2
Post High School, First Job and Conversion

After completing high school, Dr. Paul Radier who was the Chief Engineer with the Ministry of Works helped in securing the job. I got my first job as a clerical officer with the Ministry of Works in Kisumu. The job was twenty miles away from home. We all walked to and from work. It was

fun because we were always in a group. There was no set time for exercise. I carried cooked food to work. During lunchtime, my coworkers and I would sit together and share food. It was fun and exciting. At the end of the day, we all would walk back to our apartments. I never watched what I ate. Exercise or going to the gym was not part of my vocabulary. As I remember, there were no gyms. However, there was Y.W.C.A.

A year later, I had a short marriage and had two daughters. It was during the painful and traumatic events of separation and divorce that I sort more

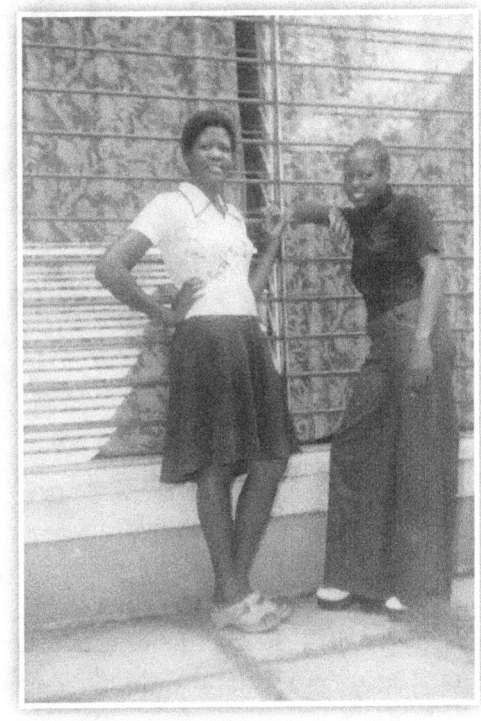

to my life. I was going to be the first woman in my whole village to separate from her husband. This was a taboo. An old friend from High school invited me to Nairobi Pentecostal church. My background was Seventh Day Adventist Church (SDA) where the pastor prays and everyone is quiet. On that Tuesday night, November 10, 1981, everyone was praying and crying to their God.

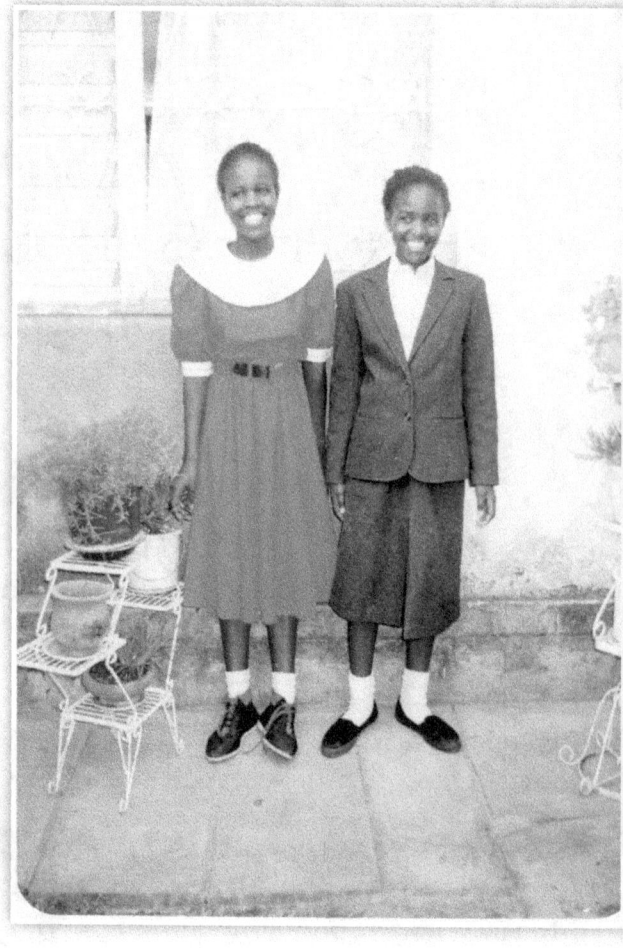

I opened my mouth and said loud 'God, *if you are there somewhere, please come into my heart and make me feel like living again'*. As soon as I finished that prayer, it felt like a load of one hundred kilogram of sugar just dropped from my head. I came to know the Lord Jesus personally on November 10, 1981. This happened a week after taking my girls to live with my mother in the rural area at Wire Village in Oyugis.

I prayed these three prayers: 1) that I would go to heaven (I did not know at the time that was part of the package) 2) that I would be a missionary someday somewhere, 3) that I would go back to school in either India or America.

I resigned from my job with the Ministry of Works and went back to school. At the Kenya Polytechnic, I studied Business Management and Secretarial. Justina Muchura, a friend of mine offered me her servant's quarter to live in while attending college. Kenya Polytechnic was within walking distance from where I lived. I did not worry about keeping fit or going to the gym. I had a small kerosene stove for cooking and cooked on very rare occasions. I bought mostly fruits and cooked vegetables when I had time. I was in shape and spent most of my time either in college or in church. I ate when angry. I had no television so I would go to bed around 9:00 pm or earlier.

I graduated from Kenya Polytechnic two years later and got my first job with FOCUS-Kenya. My job was walking to the post office, duplicating materials, and general typing. Ufungamano, where the office was located was ten miles from the city center. I would walk back and forth with no problem. This was part of my exercise. I did not even think about exercising. Ufungamano had a cafeteria, which served only fresh cooked food. We could also choose fruits or milk.

After three years working with FOCUS-Kenya, I changed jobs. I worked for Daystar University, Sudan Interior Mission (SIM), Open Doors with Brother Andrew and World Vision. I walked most of the time. This helped me keep in good shape. I was not particular about what I ate, but most foods were fresh from the garden. All foods were natural. I ate no processed foods or anything with preservatives.

I continued to work at World Vision International. I reached the top of any promotion I could get as an Administrative Assistant. I decided to enroll for French classes for more job opportunities. United Nations bodies required second or third language speakers. I wanted a better paying job to support my two daughters and myself.

Time passed and I continued with my life as a Christian, raising my two daughters, going to church, teaching Sunday school and being involved with the Women's Ministry. A number of things happened that prompted me think of going back to school. My two younger brothers died suddenly of short illnesses in 1993-1994 and my ex-husband formally did a church wedding with his second wife. I thought of the family responsibilities that would be on my shoulders.

I had been praying and waiting for my ex-husband to change his mind so that we could be remarried again. However, after fourteen years of praying and waiting, I got a distressing call from him saying he wanted my blessings to do a church wedding with his second wife. At this point, I knew there was no hope or reconciliation. I had to move on with my life.

CHAPTER 3

Preparation to come to America

During our weekly meeting at Nairobi Pentecostal Church with my dear friend Elizabeth Jacca, I shared with her my passion to go back to school. She suggested going to America to study. I liked the idea, prayed about it, and shared with my family, who were supportive. In the meantime, I wrote to one of my former bosses from World Vision International, Dr. Stephen Githumbi who at that time was a doctoral student at Fuller Theological Seminary in Pasadena, California. He visited Kenya in December 1994 and brought me applications for Biola University in La Mirada, California. I had not heard of Biola, but trusted Dr. Githumbi's choice.

I did not fill out applications for any other universities or colleges. I thought that going back to school would give me better opportunities and I would need to depend on anybody for financial support. My health was great, but I thought of pressures which, if I did not monitor, might lead to other complications. I had a good social network, but many times, I felt overwhelmed with the family demands. This put a lot of strain on my health, but I tried not to let anyone notice.

It was during the process of preparing to come to the US that I felt very tired and fainted in an elevator. Some people thought I had a phobia. Some Good Samaritan took me to hospital. The doctor advised me that I needed to slow things down. I told him there was no time and the pressure was just too much. I had three weeks to sort things out and leave the country to a place I have never been before.

Things moved very quickly with processing the application, raising money, and getting a visa to come to the United States. Raising enough money to put down as partial payment to Biola University was a struggle.

Dr. and Mrs. McMillan Kiiru helped a great deal with two fundraisings. Dr. Theuri and his family also contributed significant amount of money towards my education. Mrs. Nkita Arao, Daystar Registrar also contributed and supported me all the way. I had so much support from friends, former colleagues, my pastor, Dr. Gichinga, his late wife Emmi, family members and the whole village. The spirit of togetherness (hara- mbee) is so evident when one is in need. The late Mr. Mjema, a close friend of my late brother Sami donated one million Kenya Shillings. This was very impressive to many people.

People in Kenya see a person going to school as an advantage to the whole community. I was able to raise enough money, sold some of my belongings including books, music, furniture and the house to raise enough money for visa payment, down payment to Biola University and a one-way air ticket as a student.

My plan was to come to the US, study psychology and go back to support women who have been discriminated by men and society believing that every divorce — was a woman's fault!

I had less than three weeks to do all the final touches and leave the country. I pondered about a number of things: i) going to a new place with one-way ticket, ii) I had been out of school for over ten years. I thought of the high risk I was about to take. My heart and mind had mixed emotions.

I was excited that I was going back to school and would eventually wear a gown and a hood. I had yearned to possess a degree for a long, long time. I was also terrified: How would I make it alone in a foreign land, over ten thousand miles away? A number of thoughts crossed my mind. Suppose I do not fit in, suppose I do not understand what the teachers will be teaching? Well, I did not have enough time to process all these fears.

My eating habits also changed. I heard stories of rich U.S. foods and I was trying to find foods which would be equivalent to the U.S.'s.

During the preparation, I would walk to most places soliciting money from friends and relatives for my fundraising. I walked during that three-week period more than I ever walked in an entire year. I lost a lot of weight during this time as well. While walking from office to office, I did not have time to eat. I would only eat at the end of the day at home. By this time, we had television so we could watch some programs and still went to bed by 9:00 pm. There was only one channel — Kenya Broadcasting Corporation (KBC) controlled by the government. Going to bed early helped me keep my weight stable.

CHAPTER 4

Arrival at LAX and Biola days

The time finally came to leave my beloved country. I left Kenya on September 2, 1995 from Nairobi, Jomo Kenyatta International Airport. I boarded Royal Dutch KLM 878 to Amsterdam-Los Angeles and reached LAX on Labor Day, September 3, 1995, losing one day.

I was terrified of flying, and during the flight I made this urgent prayer to God, that if He was ready to take me home, I would prefer that He take me from the ground. I meant every word of that prayer!

I could not even eat or go to the bathroom for fear of the plane landing or something happening while I was in the bathroom. I thought of being more than thirty thousand miles above sea level and a number of thoughts crossed my mind again. I tried to relax or sleep but I could not. There was plenty of food during all the flights. I started seeing the rich foods of America. I just could not fathom how much food was served on the airplane. I said to myself, "Wooh, I am already in the land of abundance and opportunity."

My thoughts were far reaching. I thought my plane might crash. I imagined the pilot misreading his maps direction and going to a different country. I was not able to sleep for 48 hours straight. Previously, I had travelled to other parts of Kenya as well as neighboring countries, but always with ground transportation.

Coming to America and flying for twenty-four hours was a nightmare! The flight from Nairobi to Amsterdam was ten hours. I had ten hours layover in Amsterdam then I flew from Amsterdam to Minneapolis for another ten hours.

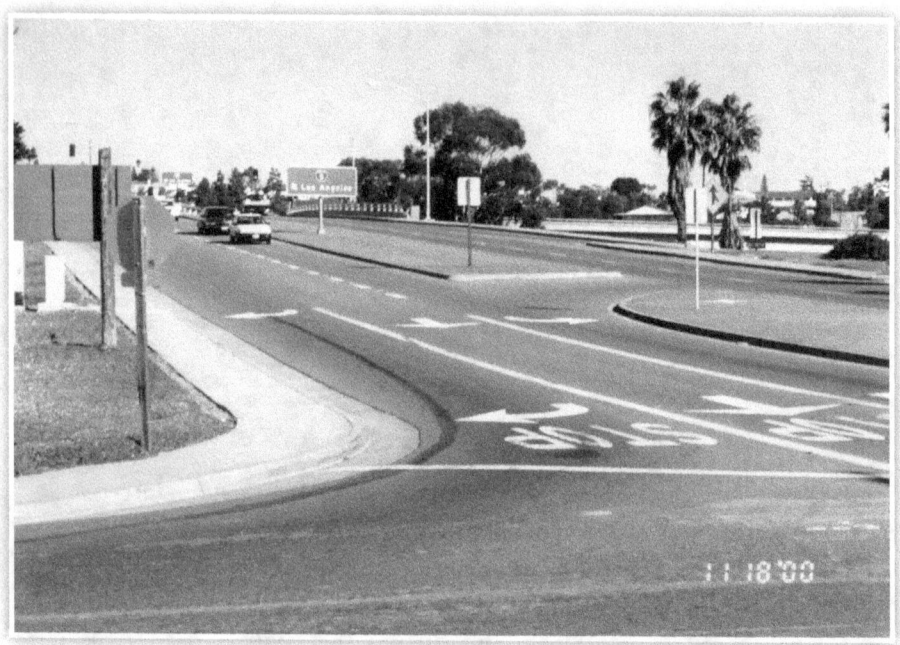

Turbulent winds in Minneapolis prevented me from making a connecting flight and I waited in the cold at Minneapolis airport, a big drop in temperature. Kenya is a tropical country. I was cold!

Finally, after a four-hour flight, I made it to Los Angeles California. By this time, I was hungry. I did not have any money to buy food and I would not have known which food to choose.

Coming to the United States for the first time was a great shock for me. I thought that coming here, as an adult it would be easier to adjust. When I arrived, I was disoriented.

I am truly grateful to God for His mercies that are new every morning and that He brought me safely to the U.S.

When I landed at LAX on September 3, 1995, I was surprised to see so many white people in one place at the same time. I was not able to distinguish between Caucasians, Latinos and other ethnicities. I could only see fair-skinned people. I thought, "Gee! Are their different colors in this part of the world?" I saw only one color of people-white.

I thought I was losing my mind or eyesight. I thought of home, family, friends, and my two daughters whom I left in the care of my sisters, and thought, "What I was doing in Los Angeles?" I still did not have an appetite.

Even today, sixteen years later, I still shudder when I think of my arrival in Los Angeles. I panicked. The International student's leader was scheduled to pick me up. I wondered if she would recognize me. I had described to her that I would be wearing a traditional African green dress with green headband with long braided hair, and no jewelry. As soon as I reached the ground, Marie Pezzota President of Biola's International Students Organization recognized me. She said, *'Welcome Betty.'* I had a sigh of relief!

My long journey had just begun. Marie drove me to the Biola University dormitory, to start my studies in the U.S. I arrived on Monday, which was a holiday-Labor Day. My roommate Lilly was a Taiwanese graduate student who had prepared a special meal for me. I could not eat because I had lost my appetite. I also did not recognize what kind of food she offered me. I felt the world was going round and round. I had to put my thoughts together quickly. I was not sure if people understood what was going on my mind. I had to go to class the following day. Classes had been in session for two weeks and on my first day, I was already two weeks behind in my classwork On top of all these, I had not been a student in over ten years.

Sharon Tortora was in one of my classes and she reached out to me. She was off campus student. She invited me to her grandmother's house, which was close to school. She also helped me with class notes to catch up for missed weeks. We still maintain that friendship even today.

I left a comfortable home in Kenya and came to U.S. to study. At that moment, I was not sure, if leaving home was a bright idea. Coming to Biola and living in a dormitory with a shared room was another shock. I had my own house in Nairobi with a personal bathroom. I felt jet lagged and did not feel like eating for a couple of days.

Another shocking incident: I went to use the bathroom at night and as soon as I walked in, the lights turned on. I quickly ran back to my room think- ing someone was hiding in there. I went back the second time and the same thing happened. I went and asked my roommate to go with me to the bathroom. She asked me why, and I told her that someone was in there. She smiled and said that bathroom was equipped with a motion sensor light. I was relieved to know that someone was not there to attack me at night.

Of course, Biola had door passes so that no outsider could enter, but that did not cross my mind at that time. I thought of night runners in Kenya.

One of the challenges that I had to face was to compete with girls my daughters' ages. I had to stay up late to catch up with my class readings and assignments. This affected my health. I was thirty-five years when I started my bachelor's degree. I had to work extra hard to compete with recent young high schools graduates.

Working many hours, studying day and night, I never had time for exercise or enough sleep, which affected my weight tremendously. I gained a lot of weight during my first two years at Biola.

Of course, I cannot forget the goodness of the Lord, which came through in different ways. I had one individual who sponsored me for the last two years at Biola. Whittier Hills Baptist Church also sponsored me for three years with Church Matching Grant. Sandy Weaver, Director of Finance department was very compassionate to me. Financial stresses were heavy on me at the beginning of each semester. I was uncertain whether I would continue. This affected my health emotionally, financially and physiologically. Fortunately, I had close prayer group partners. Kenya Interdenominational Christian Church (KICC), Mrs. Pealina Gichuhi was one of

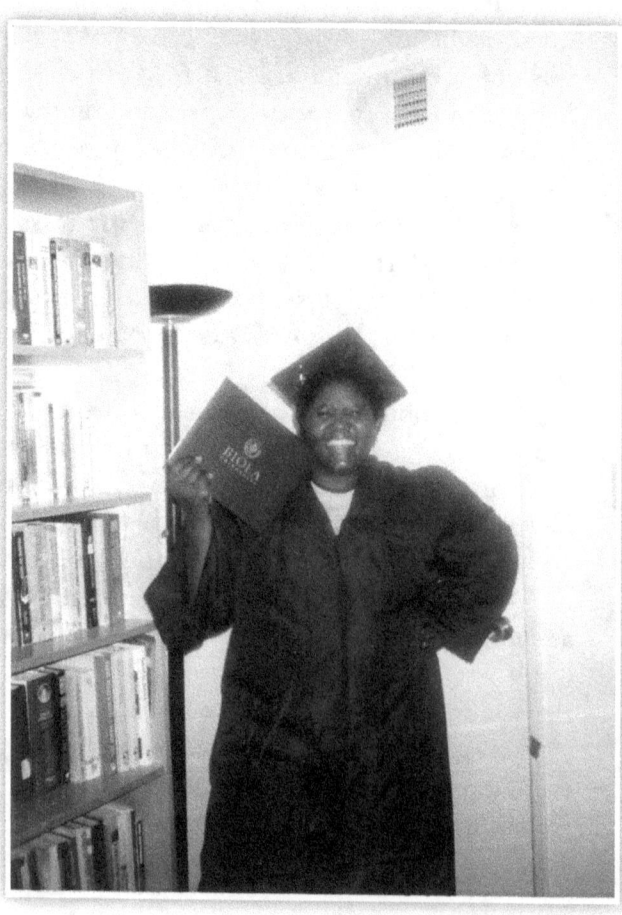

those people who prayed with me every semester. She also provided food for me during school holidays. I stayed in the dorm when everyone went home.

I finally said to myself "I can do all things through Christ who strengthens me". I also believed that I could do anything when I put my heart and mind to the task. Indeed this came true with time. I graduated from Biola University in December 1999 with a BA in psychology and minors in Sociology and Bible. Praise God!

CHAPTER 5

Moving Off Campus
and Multiple Surgeries

In April 1998, during my third year at Biola, I had to move off campus because my two daughters were coming for a visit from Kenya. I had to look for an apartment to rent. It needed to be close to school so that I could walk to school since I did not own a car. My four jobs were on campus. I was a Resident Assistant in Hart Hall 1996-1997. I worked in the cafeteria, as well as Biola Organizational Leadership Department (BOLD) and Physical Plant. On one occasion at the Physical Plant, Mashburn building, I sat for one minute and fell asleep. Martha, the supervisor found me a sleep and was kind enough not to let me go. She gave me a warning. Like many single parents, work and school became my husband. I had no time for exercise, let alone go to the gym. I also did not watch what I ate. I gained a tremendous amount of weight during this time. Cafeteria food was free and there was a large variety of food choices. We would go to places like Home Town Buffet, which was a great treat. We would eat as much as we could for only eight dollars. What a delicacy I thought!

After I moved off campus, I had to quit my on campus jobs. All my three off campus jobs were in-group homes. My physical activity level was low. During my work hours, I was sitting down, eating, driving or talking with the teenagers. I slept at my apartment once a week. I had to work at different group homes from 7am-3p, then another one from 3:30pm-10pm then work a night shift from 10:30pm to 6:00 am. I barely had time to take a shower and rush off to the next job.

By 2000, I was weighing two hundred and ninety ninety-two pounds (292). I did not even realize that I was carrying that much weight. I was still able to find clothes that fit because there were plus size clothes in many departmental stores like Ross Dress for Less or the Plus Size Store. Being heavy and finding clothes was not a problem.

In August 2000, I enrolled in graduate school at Hope International University in Fullerton. This was another very stressful time for me. I was a graduate student, had three jobs, and to balance all these with family matters, my weight soared. Weighing two hundred and ninety two (292) pounds put a lot of pressure on my heart. I did not realize how heavy I was.

My three jobs were working for different Group Homes for abused and neglected children. My two other jobs were house cleaning and occasional babysitting for families and churches. The night job was not physically engaging. I was mostly sitting down doing paperwork, doing laundry and cooking, then eating to keep awake.

I did not feel anything different about my weight except I would feel very tired after a short walk or climbing the stairs. I went to the doctor who pre- scribed medication for elevated blood pressure. I ate when I was tired. I also ate for comfort. Many low income or single mothers can identify with what it means to have 3-4 jobs. Being a graduate student, while balancing family life took all my energy.

With every pound gained, I developed all sorts of medical complications. These were high blood pressure, high cholesterol and later developed diabetes. My turning point was when I was diagnosed with diabetes.

Below is the chart for all surgeries done for hernia

Date	Hospital	Reason
9/22/2000	Fullerton Outpatient	Umbilical hernia
4/1/2002	Whittier Inpatient	Ventral-with mesh
8/12/2004	Covina Emergency	Ventral –repaired previous
12/1/2005	Whittier Inpatient	Ventral – repaired previous
3/17/2007	Redlands Emergency	Ventral-repaired bowel perforation
2/18/2011	Fontana Emergency	Ventral-another mess placed

The weight on my body made my umbilical cord big enough that it required surgery. This was the first of five hernia surgeries that followed years later.

A year after I graduated from Biola University, I went for a regular checkup and the doctor said I had umbilical hernia that needed repair and surgery. By this time, I had gained over seventy pounds. With all the six (6) hernia surgeries that followed over the next eleven years, my body became weak with lots of fatty acids and scar tissues. Each of these doctors advised me to lose weight. Of course, I tried a diet two weeks after leaving the doctor's office, but got back to my routine as soon as I was comfortable.

I was under a lot of pressure. With job demands, graduate studies and two daughters in college, I didn't have time for exercise. I was wrong! Coping with stress and demands of daily life led to an unhealthy lifestyle and an unhealthy body.

I had had an extended belly button when I was a child and it did not bother me. As an adult, my belly button had significantly extended outward, and developed umbilical hernia. When the doctor suggested that I needed an operation, I agreed. The doctor indicated that it would be an outpatient procedure and I should be able to go back to normal duties within a week or two.

This was my first hernia repair. Surgery was scheduled on September 22, 2000. I was terrified when I arrived at the Hospital in Fullerton for the first hernia surgery. My blood pressure was elevated to 200/150 and the doctor said he could not perform the surgery with that kind of blood pressure because it was too risky. I called a couple friends of mine who were also attendees of Whittier Hills Baptist Church to pray with me. Arlene and Bill Dalton came to the Hospital in Fullerton and prayed.

As soon as they finished praying, the high blood pressure dropped to 130/90. To the doctor and me it was one of those instant miracles. The doctor performed the surgery after the drop in blood pressure. Four hours later, my best friend Iris Kidula took me home.

The recovery time was longer than one week as the doctor had predicted. I stayed home for another five weeks, which effected my work hours, money, and income. I had not worked long enough to qualify for vacation time or paid leave. The thought of not being able to pay for my bills, school and other necessities increased my stress and eating habits. I ate anything and everything. I am not sure I was depressed but my financial needs were great. My blood pressure increased and medication was unable to control it.

After getting well, I continued working 3-4 jobs along with graduate school at Hope International University in Fullerton for a Master's degree. At this point, the financial pressures were four times greater. Being a graduate student, having two kids in college with no employment or even eligible for employment was too much to handle. When things were too emotionally difficult to handle, I resorted to food, and of course, I did not control the portions or the type of food I ate. As an international student, there are many restrictions in terms of getting jobs, school loans etc. I had to work many hours to put myself through college and graduate school and to pay for my kids' college education as well.

With every pound I gained, the increased weight brought more health complications. I had a second hernia surgery on April 1, 2002. Prior to this, I had constant pain on my lower abdomen. I was a second year student at Hope International University at this time. I went for a checkup and the doctor confirmed that I had a ventral hernia that needed repair and surgery. My primary doctor referred me to a surgeon at Whittier. I remember sharing the upcoming surgery with my classmates at Hope and the professor mentioned that he had had a hernia repaired when he was in high school and he never had any problems with it again. That professor encouraged me to have the hernia repaired.

The doctor said, my recovery time would be 2-4 weeks. During Easter break, I had the operation. Iris Kidula drove me to the hospital. This time I was not scared but I was terrified of the anesthetist. The anesthetist did not talk. He pushed the mask to my mouth. I tried to remove it and he said with a harsh tone, "What are you doing?" I did not fall asleep quickly. I could hear the lead surgeon and my doctor talking except I did not understand what they were saying. I finally became torpid and the surgery was performed. After surgery, they took me to the recovery room. My friend Iris was already waiting there. I could not recognize her. She and everyone around her looked like tress. I was hallucinating. She told me later that she called my name and I could not respond. After several hours in recovery room, I was taken to my room.

I had not seen the marks on my stomach, and when I saw eight cuts with bandages on them, I went into shock. My blood pressure elevated to 190/102.

The nurses rushed to my room and asked what the problem was. I told them, that my doctor had not explained prior to surgery about the eight cuts on my stomach. The nurse paged the doctor, and he came two hours later. He explained that the surgery was laparoscopic with mesh. I could not reverse the cuts, but I had to accept the eight marks on my stomach. I stayed in the hospital for five days for observation.

Iris took me home upon discharge. God bless her. I had never felt so much pain in my entire life. One of the incisions, started to bleed. I went back to the surgeon who was not very sympathetic. He blamed me for not taking care of the wounds and being obese.

Two months later, I went back to him because of the pain and his response was "I was paid for surgery by your insurance, not for pain man-

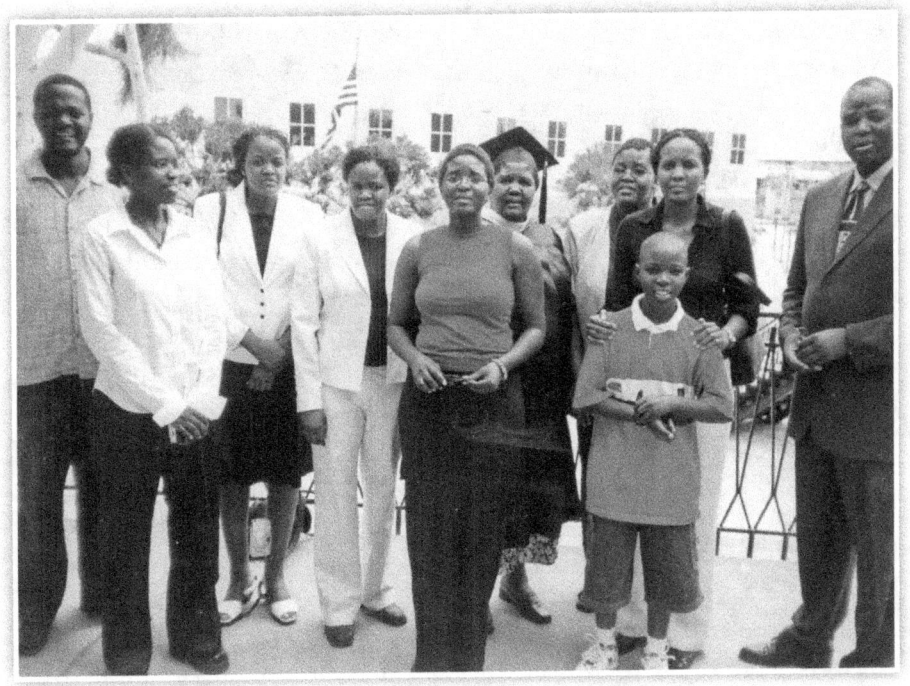

agement". He reiterated that my weight was preventing the healing of the surgery wounds.

There was a great financial demand with graduate school and two kids in college. Being a single parent and the sole provider, there was no time to worry about exercises or getting in shape. I had to maintain and keep three jobs at all times to keep us out of financial ruin.

During this time, losing weight was not a priority in my life. Watching my weight or going to the gym or any kind of workout/exercise was of little concern to me. I am truly grateful to God for His provisions and mercies that are new every day. In May 2003, I graduated from Hope International University in Fullerton, CA with a MA in Psychology.

I continued working at San Gabriel Children's Center (SGCC). One day I was driving to work on La Mirada Blvd and someone, rear-ended my car. First, I thought it was an earthquake, which is common in California. I had stopped at a stop sign waiting for the road to be clear. I could not move from my car. Someone called 911. The paramedics checked and examined me. They asked if they could transport me to a hospital and I declined. I called my supervisor and he told me to wait for him. He came and dropped me at my house. The car was a total wreck and was towed away.

During the next two weeks, I was in bed with back and neck pain. As I was lying in bed, my eating habits did not improve. I ate the wrong foods out of frustration because I was missing time from work and receiving no pay. I gained even more pounds during that time. I was miserable and very unhappy inside.

A year after I graduated from Hope International School, life continued as usual until my visit to the doctor who said I needed a third hernia repair and surgery. I ignored him. On August 12, 2004, I was working at San Gabriel Children's Center at the time as a Clinician. We had auditors coming that week and I decided to stay in the office late to finish my clinical notes. After 11:30 pm, I left the office and headed to the parking lot. I had been sitting for many hours that day. The doctor had advised to move around every 2-3 hours.

I got into my car and felt a very sharp pain in my abdomen. I could not move and vomited all over the place. I sat in my car for a long time until one of the night supervisors was doing her rounds and saw me in my car. She came in and found me lying on the chair. Her name was Silvia She made a quick decision and rushed me to a nearby hospital Emergency Room.

Upon arriving at the ER, the doctors did an x-ray and determined that I needed an immediate hernia repair and surgery again. I asked them to contact my primary physician. I was not able to talk to him, but the ER doctor said, my doctor gave them the okay to go ahead with the surgery. This time, I was not under any normal anesthesia. They injected my spinal code with anesthesia, which was extremely painful. During the operation, the doctor put a cover in front of my face so I could not see them perform surgery, but I heard every word and the sound of the needles. The surgery took four hours. Later I transferred to a recovery room, then to my room.

During my stay at the hospital, I was nauseated and vomited and the sutures came loose. The doctor had to suture them again. Again, I was not under any anesthesia and it was very painful. I stayed in the hospital for three days. My col- leagues from San Gabriel Children's Center (SGCC) including my office mate Katie came to see me and brought me flowers and get-well cards made by my clients. This was very touching and helped me recover faster.

I resumed my busy work schedule after this. In October 5, 2004, my primary physician referred me to a gynecologist for something he explained could be a fibroid that needed surgery. I went for lab test that revealed that I had an enlarged uterus with multiple uterine fibroid. The gynecologist explained that removing the fibroid would reduce the chances of uterine cancer in the future when I reach menopause. He also explained that during the surgery, he would remove my uterus and cervix depending on the procedure. He explained that this would put me into menopause and no chance I would have more children.

The surgery was scheduled on October 21, 2004 at 7:00 am. Upon arrival, the nurse gave me a hospital gown. I walked into the changing room, panicked, and left the hospital and drove back to my apartment. I do not remember how I did it, but I did. Upon reaching home, I called the hospital and told them that I panicked and did not want my uterus removed. I was still hopeful and trusted God to be able to have more children. The gynecologist was not angry with me. The doctor responded by stating, "It is fine; we will do the surgery when you are ready." I was relieved!

I was also worried about the recovery time because I did not want to lose hours from work.

I continued to work at San Gabriel Children's Center. On December I, 2005, I had a fourth hernia surgery. After the third surgery in 2004, I was constantly in pain. I could not sleep on my stomach, or my back. I could not do any exercise without feeling extreme pain. I was miserable and made yet another appointment to see the doctor. The doctor said, the hernia needed another repair and surgery. My heart was broken. I could not understand how I could go for so many surgeries for the same thing. I called my mother in Kenya and asked her to support me in prayer again. She finally had the courage to ask, "Aren't their qualified American doctors who can do the surgery once and for all?" This particular doctor mentioned that the first hernia surgery with mesh was not done correctly.

This time, I was terrified again, not because of the doctor, but the process on anesthesia. I have a phobia on anesthetists. My older daughter drove me to the hospital for surgery. When the anesthetist came, he asked me how long I had had a Pace Maker. I was shocked because I had never had a pacemaker put on my heart. He looked at the chat again and found out that the particular report was switched with someone else's.

My blood pressure and heart rate was rising. I asked to see the surgeon. The doctor came into the room and assured me that he would operate on the right place. I was not convinced. I had seen in many movies where incorrect operations done on the wrong patient and the patient's charts being misplaced or switched.

My imagination went wild. My daughter assured me but that was not good enough. I asked the doctor to draw with a pen where the surgery will be done- and he did on my stomach.

A few minutes later, I was taken to the surgery room. I could not fall asleep. I kept on thinking that there might be another mix-up and they might operate on my head instead of my stomach. The surgeon came one hour later and I was still awake. The operating team responded that I could not fall asleep.

After seeing my doctor, I was assured that all would be well and finally I fell asleep. The surgery was done. It took five hours. The surgery was done on December 2, 2005.

I stayed home for two months recovering. Upon returning to my job at San Gabriel Children's Center (SGCC), the company was going through financial strains. I was transferred to a lower level. I was not happy but I could not do anything because they had petitioned for my HI-B visa and I had to stick with them. In April 2006, I just could not take it anymore. I shared this with a good friend of mine, Dr. Finnian Ebuehi, a former colleague and classmate who had prayed with me on many occasions.

CHAPTER 6

Weight Gain and Medical Complications

In 2005, my highest weight was two hundred and ninety three (293) pounds. I was only seven pounds shy of 300 pounds. I had a Body Mass Index of 47.9. My height and body structure made me carry the weight in all the right places.

That same year, one of my brothers, who knew I was struggling with my weight, sent me Hoodia tablets. These tables originated in Southern Africa. This highly advertised fast type of weight loss product was on the market, though not approved by the Food and Drug Administration (FDA). It claimed to be an appetite suppressant and could help with weight loss.

During that time, I was on many medications and decided to consult with my primary doctor. The doctor reacted by stating, "If you know someone overweight and you don't like them, give it to them." I never took the tablets; neither did I give them to anyone else.

In March of 2006, I bought my first home in Redlands, CA. While dropping some item at the Goodwill Store, my brakes failed and I ran into a stopped truck.

Both my daughters were in the car with me. The car caught fire because of impact and was totaled. All of us were safe, thank God. I had problems with my insurance company who refused to pay, stating that collision was not included. I had just paid off $24,000.00 after four years for my Toyota Camry. This brought more stress. I was moving to a new home, taking a new job and now I had no car!

I comforted myself by eating the wrong foods and not taking care of myself. I did not have time for exercise or to go to the gym. I rented a car for one month before getting one of my own. I missed a couple of other payments. My credit score dropped to below 600, which affected my purchase of a used car, which made the interest rocket up to be 14%. Food was a comfort to me. I was very angry with my insurance company. I had paid my insurance religiously for over ten years without any accident. I was disappointed that, the insurance company did not help when I needed them the most. I ate for comfort and was not exercising regularly.

In April 2006, I tendered my resigned from San Gabriel Children's Center and joined the David and Margaret Home, in La Verne. I was a Residential Therapist for a cottage of six girls. I enjoyed and loved my work. D&M had a gym on campus. I took it upon myself to take at least two girls who were doing well in the cottage for workouts. This helped a bit, but my eating habits were still bad.

I worked many hours and ate the wrong foods whenever I was hungry. After two years, I was transferred to the Mental Health Department, where my duties allowed me to sit while doing therapy. I gained over thirty pounds in three months in this department.

In November of 2006, I joined LA Fitness and engaged a personal trainer for one year. This was quite expensive. By that time, I weighed 280 pounds with a Body Mass Index of 43.8. After one year, I lost 30 pounds and gained 30+after I stopped working out with the personal trainer. It was too costly to continue with a personal trainer. My monthly payment plus membership was five hundred and twenty dollars ($520.00). I continued to go to the gym, at least 3-4 times a week, but my eating habits were still poor.

By this time, I was on three different medications for High blood pressure and two for high cholesterol. One side effect of these pills was weight gain. I stopped losing weight.

Prior to surgery on January 15, 2007, I was in so much pain that I had to call 911. My younger daughter was living with me at the time. The ambulance rushed me to Loma Linda Hospital. The CAT scan showed that I had inflamed bowel. The doctors at Loma Linda suggested that I go to my primary physician for more observation and tests. I felt better after a few weeks and did not follow up until two months later when the pain came back again. I was rushed to ER again.

On March 7, 2007. I woke up with a lot of pain in my lower abdomen. I could not move fast. I did not want to call in sick from work, so I decided to drive slowly to La Verne to my job at D&M. Upon my arrival, the pain increased. I told one of the staff members, that I was not feeling well. I was not able to attend the staff meeting. I lay on the couch and could not move. I thought I was dying. I could not breathe and I was in tremendous pain. I dialed the staff extension and told Rosemary, one of the staff, that I was not feeling well.

She asked if I needed an a ambulance, but I responded that I did not want to alarm the whole campus with ambulance siren. Rosemary acted quickly upon seeing my condition and called for an ambulance. The paramedics were on campus within ten minutes. They examined me and decided to transport me to the nearest hospital. Rosemary and Marlene stayed with me at the hospital.

The doctor performed the tests. The X-rays and CAT scan on my abdomen led to a diagnosis of an Infraumbilical hernia. After being at the hospital for an hour, the doctor came to my room and said, "I will be performing your surgery. Get ready."

"Ok," I said, and had a flashback of the two previous anesthetists whom I feared before my two previous surgeries. I panicked and called the nurse in charge. I told her that I wanted to be transported to Redlands and see my own doctor before the surgery, or my doctor could refer me to another surgeon in Redlands, which was closer to my home.

The nurse said she could not make that decision and called the doctor. The doctor explained that my condition was serious and they could not take a chance of releasing me from the hospital. The doctor asked me to sign a release that I refused medical advice. The doctor explained to the nurse and put on my chart that his impression was my condition was an incarcerated recurrent ventral incisional hernia.

The plan was exploratory laparotomy and repair of the recurrent ventral incisional hernia with possible bowel resection.

My younger daughter came and drove me to our home in Redlands. I did not go to the hospital that night and decided to sleep at home hoping the pain would go away. The pain never did. I was miserable the whole night. In the morning, I called my primary physician who suggested I get an ambulance to ER immediately. The ambulance took me to the Community Hospital and I was admitted for surgery.

On March 17, 2007, I had a fifth hernia surgery. The surgeon explained to me that the recurrences of the hernia were related to being over- weight. I knew this and did not want a reminder. Upon admission at the hospital, my weight was 285. I was on six different medications.

The surgery could not take place immediately because my potassium level was too low. I had a potassium transfusion before the surgery was done. For some reason, I felt comfortable with the surgeon. My primary physician, also came to see me before the surgery. He assured me that I was in safe hands. I trusted him. My doctor was overweight himself so he never pushed me to lose weight during my office visits with him.

I had struggles with my weight after coming to America. I tried four different weight loss programs. Two of them worked for about six months, but I gained the original weight plus twenty-five pounds more. This was very discouraging. I almost went through depression but bounced back to life. Some people might feel offended but being over forty and over weight is not a good combination if you are looking for a job.

Whether we like it or not, many people respond negatively to over-weight people.

I continued working at the David and Margaret Home. My employer D&M Home changed health coverage to Kaiser Permanente. I made my first appointment on January 4, 2008 and met with a doctor whom I admired and immediately connected with him. My weight was 274 pounds! My blood pressure was 138/75. The doctor's office gave me a print out about Body Mass Index (BMI) which is a number that measures both your weight and height. The nurse explained that it is a good way to understand the effect of my weight and health. I am 5'7". A BMI of 30 or more put me at HIGHER RISK for weight health problems resulting from my excess weight. My weight greatly increased my chances for high blood pressure, diabetes, heart disease, stroke, arthritis, breathing and sleeping problems, some types of cancer, and even depression. Knowing my BMI level helps me want to change my eating and physical activity habits in an effort to to avoid weight gain while lowering my health risks.

In August 2008, I continued with LA Fitness gym club and hired a personal trainer again. I continued with this for one year and lost twenty pounds. The loss was not significant enough to impact noticeable body changes. The doctor insisted I still needed to lose more weight. The thought of spending more time attempting to lose more weight, and the stress this brought, made me eat wrong food and not want to exercise.

On the morning of April 9 2009, I felt very tired at work at the D&M Home. I shared with my immediate supervisor, Paula R., who was kind enough to make sure I was feeling better. I went to the company's nurse who checked my blood pres- sure and it was 180/105. She suggested I go to the doctor or emergency room immediately. Instead, I drove home to get some rest. Upon arriving at home, I found a very unpleasant situation that increased my blood pressure. After about twenty minutes at home, I was not feeling too well. Finally went to the doctor and was I admitted for observation.

My blood pressure was 190/120, which greatly concerned my doctor. I stayed for two days and the blood pressure stabilized. This is when the doctors also found that my hernia had elongated and needed to be repaired for the sixth time. I was not ready for another hernia surgery and asked the doctor to release me to go home. I went back home and consulted with my primary physician who also confirmed that the hernia needed repair again. Up to this point, I had had five operations for the same hernias repair and surgeries. I finally got well and life continued as normal.

January of 2009, I had to go back to school to keep my immigration status current and legal. I started a PhD program at Alliant International University in Alhambra, CA. This created another stressful situation. I was now working in a PhD program. I had to be a full time student to qualify for immigration status and I had three jobs. I had to quit my job at Guardians of Love, San Bernardino, CA, and at that time, my house was going in a foreclosure. I had too many external stressors.

My immediate supervisor Paula and Michael were very understanding and supportive. I could not thank them enough! The classes were three days a week and she agreed that I could schedule my hours and therapy time with the clients around my free times. I still do not know how I managed but I barely did. I was not able to get any student loans as an international student. I used all my savings to pay for the first semester. Unfortunately, I only managed to go to school for two semesters. I had classes on Monday, Wednesday and Thursday from 3:00pm-10pm. I lived two hours away from school and one hour away from work. The stress of driving and traffic on the freeways was almost unbearable. I somehow barely managed. Of course, I was on five different medications. Of course, my weight was still too high, I weighed two hundred and eighty (280) pounds.

While traveling to South Bend- Indiana on June 28, 2009 for a live Radio TV Show with The Harvest Show, I sat next to a woman who was very amiable. We were in a very small plane from Atlanta to Indiana. When the flight attendant announced that people should put their seat belts, I mentioned to this woman that every time I travel, I tell myself that I will lose weight so that the seat belt can go round my waist without pushing in my stomach. The woman responded, "Do you really want to lose weight"?

I affirmatively said "YES!" After landing, she introduced me to her 'Health Coach' Marianne Garrett. She gave me her card and a few days, later after returning to California, I called her to check on the program that helps people lose and maintain weight.

Of course, I had tried, several weight loss programs and I was skeptical, as any of us would be.

I checked with my primary doctor before venturing into The Medifast pro- gram. I started this medically proven program on July 11, 2009. I weighed 277 pounds (23 pounds away from 300 pounds). I lost thirty (30) pounds in six months. After stopping Medifast because it was too expensive, I gained thirty plus pounds. This kind of weight gain increased my depression and despair. I also tried Jenny Craig for six months, lost 40 pounds and gained forty plus when I stopped. I also tried Dr. Atkins – all protein diet. I lost twenty pounds in four months and gained twenty plus when I stopped.

On July 8, 2009, I got a life scare experience! I was rushed to Emergency Room in an ambulance with elevated High Blood Pressure of 169/102. The doctors said it was a 'mini, mild, small stroke. The scary bit was the <u>STROKE</u> part. It appeared to me that I had a second chance in life.

Prior to this, I was involved in a lot of things including being a full time PhD student, maintaining a full time job as a Mental Health Therapist, promoting my book, working on an online magazine, and various other types of work. My motivation was to be financially stable.

CHAPTER 7
Forgetfulness

By 2009, I was on three medications for high blood pressure and two medications for high cholesterol. One of the side effects of the medications that bothered me greatly was forgetfulness. It did not occur occasionally, or for minute incidences, but it came about on several important occasions. One major incident was during my PhD courses, where I had a conference call with one of the professors. The professor had given me a very poor grade and we scheduled a phone conference to dispute it with the chairperson of the department and other professors. One would think that something that important would be impossible to forget.

I completely forgot about it until I got a phone call from the secretary. Her reaction was "Betty, we have been waiting for your call for the last twenty minutes." To make matters worse, I asked what the call was about and the reason for it. She explained that because I did not honor my promise to a conference call, my poor grade could not be changed. You can imagine the anger and rage that I felt within me. I kept asking myself, "How did I forget about the conference call?" I went to my room and found that I had written this date three times in three different places and yet, my brain could not recall it.

I started putting things together. I realized that I was becoming more forgetful. For example, I would forget where I placed my toothbrush if I had to answer a phone call.

I began scrutinizing and reading all labels and the side effects of the medications. I found that one of the blood pressure medications' side effects was forgetfulness. I made an appointment with my primary physician and shared with him how I had been forgetful. He never argued with me and said, "Yes, that is one of the side effects I will change your medication." This situation was very frustrating.

Although, doctors have a wealth of knowledge, if there is one person who knows about my body I have carried for over fifty years, it is I!

One thing that I do is to read all the labels in any medication I take including the small print. Certainly, knowing your body and noticing small changes and signs should be taken seriously.

On November 9, 2009, which was also my first daughter's birthday, my employer terminated my employment because the doctor had not released me to go back to work. The company needed someone to cover my cases. This was devastating. This employer was the one who petitioned for my green card, and I could not look for another job unless I get a new employer to petition for me for a new work authorization for employment. Nonimmigrants as the law requires, must have an employer to petition for their work authorization. A work authorization (called HI-B) is good with one employer at a time. I was now worried about my immigration status, employment, money, and insurance. My house was in foreclosure. I had family problems and I was overweight. I thought I was losing my mind.

My eating habits were horrible. I had no time to cook at home. I ate on the go most of the time.

I went to see my doctor routinely and again my blood pressure was elevated. This time it had risen up to 180/101. He was concerned about this but he assured me that things would be all right someday.

At this time, I was too proud to see a therapist about the stressful issues in my life, and I said to myself that I was a therapist and I would be my own doc- tor. I could not see things objectively. It was a very hard time for me. I thank God every day for my friend Paul S from New York, who was supportive. He would call to encourage me and just to talk from time to time. I was living alone. I ate to comfort myself. I was unhappy.

I was depressed. I called Kaiser's, behavioral department and made an appointment to see a therapist. I knew that if I did not make a quick decision, I was going to end up in a mental hospital. No matter how strong I was, the issues were too overwhelming.

I saw a male therapist, who was very kind. I cried most of the session. All these external stressors were killing me inside. I also had issues with one of my daughter's and a sister, which was an extra burden. The therapist quickly referred me to a psychiatrist.

The doctor diagnosed me as Bipolar II. I vehemently disagreed. I know how to diagnose people, and I certainly was not bipolar. He put me on two medications, Lithium and Abilify, for three days. They interacted with other medications I was taking for high blood pressure, and high cholesterol. After three days, I went back to see the doctor and he discontinued those medications.

After seeing the therapist and psychiatrist for two weeks, they assigned me a 16 weeks group session dealing with depression and social stressors. I was losing my house. I had lost my job. I had family problems, and worried about my immigration status and I had health issues. My weight continued to increase. I was not taking care of myself. I did not go to the gym. I ate for comfort and ate the wrong foods.

I was miserable and unhappy inside. On the surface, I put on a smiley face.

CHAPTER 8
Disappointments

On September 3, 2009, my 14th anniversary to the US, I got a letter from the immigration department stating that my green card process was dismissed for some technical reasons. I was distraught. My future looked bleak. I had dropped out of the PhD program. I no longer had a job, sick, depressed, and overweight, and on top of that, I no longer had prospect of getting a green card. I had stayed in the US for a long time. I did not know how to react. Going back home in Kenya was terrifying. Where would I start? I had no home in Kenya. Both my girls were here in the U.S., and I had no husband or prospects for marriage.

During ta group session, I cried the entire time. The therapist for the group asked why I was in that group. I was too emotional to respond to her immediately. After a half an hour, I shared that I am a therapist myself and on the verge of collapse. The lead therapist was very polite and kind. She made this statement, which caught my attention, "Speaking or talking about your problem may not take it away, but it surely will reduce the pain". Before completing this class, I requested a new psychiatrist. Kaiser assigned me a different doctor with whom I felt connected and comfortable. He listened to me and did not judge me. He changed the diagnosis to Major Depression Not Otherwise Specified (NOS).

I was comfortable with this diagnosis. By the end of the sixteen-week program, I finally saw a light at the end of the tunnel!

Life appeared normal again. During the month of September, I attended Redlands Home Owner's Association meeting and during our small talk, a woman by the name of Susie, invited me to their church's dinner on September 22 2009. I attended this function at Trinity Church in Redlands and fell in love with the church and the people. Pastor Paul who was the leader of this meeting (50+, though I was not fifty yet) welcomed me warmly. I have attended this church ever since. I have had much support from the women's Bible Study and the elders.

This kind of support helped me spiritually and socially. I did not share my personal struggles and baggage. I only shared about immigration matters.

I cannot thank God enough for His leading to this new church I needed to heal and God provided this church. We prayed about my immigration status. By this time, I did not have any money and could not afford an attorney. I read all the instructions for the green card application. I filled out the application and popped it in the mail. Things moved very quickly and my work permit and travel documents were approved before the end of the year. I finally got my Green Card approved in January 2011 after 16 years of waiting. I cannot thank God enough for His perfect timing.

With this one burden lifted, I could now focus on other things like working on my weight and exercising. Living in a foreign country with limited possibilities because of my immigration status, and other legal issues completely drain a person's energy.

The year 2010 was also very difficult. I willingly decided to be a foster parent for teenagers. These are court awarded children from abused and neglected backgrounds. I had four teenagers ranging from fourteen to eighteen years old. The house was a nightmare. Police were in my house almost every night. The girls would run away, fight and pick arguments with the neighbors. This stressed me out completely. I could not sleep at night in fear of one of them sneaking out of the house. I also ate very poorly. Two of the girls did not eat fish or could even stand the smell of it. Therefore, I stopped buying fish. I did not have time to go to the gym because I could not leave the girls alone. They were not yet enrolled in schools. This kind of stress increased my poor eating habits and affected my sleep pattern.

Life continued to be normal again after the foster teens left my house. I continued to see my gynecologist every year for four years, he suggested that it was a good idea to remove the fibroid tumors since they were getting bigger and made my period heavy every month. The fibroid plus other surgeries were performed on Monday January 17 2011 at 9:00 am, at Kaiser in Fontana. My doctor was there before the surgery. The anesthetist from Kaiser Permanente was very kind and I was comforted. I went to surgery without any fear at all. I stayed at the hospital one night for observation. I had no pain did I take any painkillers.

I had a lot of support from my group at Women of Trinity Bible Study. They brought me food and prayed with me. Pastor Paul and his wife also visited and prayed with me.

Well, because I had plenty of food, I ate mindlessly. I was still unhappy with unresolved issues.

CHAPTER 9

The Beginning of change & Life transformation

On February 13, 2011, I had severe pain in my lower abdomen. I could not breathe. I called a Kaiser Permanente nurse who advised me go to ER if the pain persisted. By 4:00 am, the pain was so severe that I had to call 911. The paramedics came within ten minutes and transported me to Kaiser Permanente in Fontana.

At the hospital ER, one of the doctors came and tried to push the right side of my stomach, which had protruded, and it was extremely painful. That doctor then decided that I needed another hernia surgery, and I was transferred to the main hospital for observation. The surgeon on that floor examined me and put me on liquids until he could determine what to do next.

The purpose was to have a bowel movement, which I had not had for nine days. The doctor was worried, but the nurses were aware of my condition and I was assured I was in the right place and safe. On the tenth day, the doctor decided to perform another hernia surgery. I was not terrified because I had confidence in this doctor and the anesthetist as well.

The sixth hernia surgery was done on February 18, 2011. The surgery took five hours, and then I moved to a recovery room. I was disoriented. I was transferred back to my room. I stayed there for another day and was discharged. Painkillers were prescribed. Jeanie O., leader of Women's Monday Bible study visited me and we prayed together.

My weight was affecting my health. I needed to listen to the doctor and take some action.

Over the years, I had developed these diseases: hypertension (high blood pressure, hyperlipidemia (high blood fats), obesity (BMI more than 40).

Living in a rich country like the U.S., makes people take certain things for granted. It is easy to own a car in the U.S. and there is easier access to more places by car than on foot. A few privileges make life easier. This encourages laziness. Washers and dryers, dishwashers, microwaves allow us to work less. A healthy diet can be very expensive. Fish, fruits and vegetable can be particularly overpriced. I had to cut down on sugary drinks, snacks, takeaways, and save to buy healthier foods.

Other complications I had had for a long time was indigestion and acid reflux. I had gone to many different doctors with no success. I used all kinds of indigestion and other anti-acid reflux medications. I had problems passing gas or going to the bathroom. I was constantly constipated no matter what I ate.

I was used to eating extremely fast. I could consume a full plate within 2-8 minutes. I was always in a rush even when there was no place to go.

I had to do some soul searching about my health and eating habits. I asked myself these questions: When did this eating urge start? What was going on in my life? What was I feeling or thinking? What do I really want and need now? Was I feeling angry, unloved, not valued, lonely, lethargic, afraid, worried or misplaced? Was there a feeling that I did not want to deal with right now?

Well, after going through this ordeal, I took it upon myself to read every tiny bit of side effects of any medication I was taking.

I had many things I used as excuses not to exercise. I had no time, my job was stressful, I did not feel comfortable in gym suits, or I was not good at anything. Other reasons were fear of injury, lack of interest, laziness, or not being concerned about my weight.

However, when my weight reached two hundred and eighty (280) pounds and I developed diabetes, I had to do something about it-and I did!

On many occasion, I ate when I was angry, sad or disappointed. I ate foods that were high in starch like bread, rice, or potatoes. There was a soothing sensation after eating these kinds of foods. I was eating senselessly. I was not savoring the food, but rather using it to comfort my feelings. I would feel bad and guilty but did nothing to change my feelings.

My depression partly related to eating habits. I ate when I was angry, disappointed or for emotional support. My overeating increased my depression in certain ways.

I asked myself, "Why do some people stop eating when they are full, while others continue to eat even when they are full"? My mind plays a big role in deciding whether to stop eating or not. I ate for emotional support to sooth my pain. I started losing after I separated my mind and body needs.

I learned that diabetes is not a silent killer. I read constantly about diabetes, heart disease, and other related diseases. I read that heart disease is common in people with diabetes. I also found that people with Type 2 diabetes are more prone to heart disease risks. I had high blood pressure and high cholesterol. When I was diagnosed with diabetes, it was too much for me to handle.

At this point, I was at a high risk of stroke or heart attack without any warning. I do not have a history of diabetes in my family so, I was comforted that there was a chance I could still do something about it.

Monday, February 07, 2011 9:30 am was the first day I started the Kaiser Permanente Options classes. I did not have the energy to change my lifestyle of eating, exercising and behaviors, until early 2011. I attended medical Life Options for twelve weeks and it was a great revelation. My height was 5"7" (1.702 m) with my weight at 279 lbs. (126.554 kg) at the beginning of those classes. I was very discouraged and pessimistic. I even said to myself, *"where did I go wrong that someone has to tell me how, when and what to eat"?*

I went home that day and felt depressed. I ate what I was not supposed to eat including pasta and white potatoes. I have loved bread and peanut butter for a long time and someone telling to stop was almost like someone telling me I cannot have air. After the second day, I called a Kaiser nurse to talk to her about the low calories intake. I had just bought a very expensive whole wheat bread. Her response was *"give the bread to the birds"*. I did not find that funny at the time.

In March of 2011, I felt very dizzy and thought I was having heart attack. I called 911 and was rushed to ER. The doctor confirmed that it was not a heart attack but vertigo. The doctor explained that vertigo occurs where there is a conflict between the signals sent to the brain by various balance and position sensing system of the body. The brain used four sensory systems to maintain a sense of balance.

The doctor suggested that I needed "to clear all my surroundings in my house so that I do not hit my head on something". I imagined myself as a prisoner in my own home.

The doctor also explained that nobody knows exactly why it happens, but it could be because of various muscles in the head getting extremely stiff. I had neck and shoulder pain during that visit.

The doctor gave a list of all vertigo symptoms including allergies, flu, colds, vomiting, diarrhea, fever and dehydration, rapid breathing, anxiety and stress and the use of tobacco, alcohol and illegal drugs.

She also explained that the worst case of vertigo is when all the muscles in the head work together to permanently disrupting the inner sense of balance. The doctor told me that there is no medical cure, but a few changes in diet, exercising and sleeping well could help. She prescribed over the counter medication.

Finally, the good news is after losing some weight, the feeling of vertigo disappeared. I do not feel dizzy anymore and I do not have symptoms of vertigo. What a relief!

During my twelve weeks of trainings at Kaiser Permanente Option classes, I learned that one ought to chew food thoroughly before swallowing and eat slowly 20-30 minutes each meal.

They also suggested that I do not eat and watch television at the same. I was taught to put food on a small place and not to sit next to food that is tempting when eating at home or in public.

I compared my struggle with weight loss to real life. I thought of a process for all things from the time I wake up, until I go to bed. Making decisions on which clothes to wear, what to eat for breakfast, and what to carry for lunch can be time consuming. With food, it is the process of choosing which foods to buy, what ingredients to include, and in what quantities which can be lead to success.

The process can be quite arduous, but I have learned not to analyze too much about the process-just cook it. Home-prepared meals are delicious and healthy.

It is a process to prepare food and to make it tasty and enjoyable. The more time I spend preparing, the more I will enjoy it. I agree that food prepared at home is healthier than food bought from outside. I had reasons not to prepare food at home. I argued that I had no time, no energy, not enough knowledge or just laziness. Whatever the reason, food prepared at home is the best.

With any change in my life, preparation was important. I thought of long distance and marathon runners. I had to prepare myself mentally, physically and emotionally with weight loss. I must prepare myself and commit to the changed lifestyle because it is a long process to convert my habits to healthier ones, to maintain a healthy weight loss process. Practice: This is the hardest part in life's progress. Many times, I knew what was right to eat, and yet, I choose to eat the very thing that is a pollutant to my body. My mind played tricks with me. It took me a while to discipline my mind to do what I know is good for my body.

CHAPTER 10

Weight Loss and Lifestyle Changes

By end of August 2011, I had lost thirty-six pounds (36 lbs.) and my blood sugar had dropped drastically. I went for blood work and the doctor confirmed the situation. He took me off the two medications. I have not taken those medications again. I am truly grateful for the support I had from my doctors, nurses and other non-medical people. I made these changes mostly for my health. I had a blood work done for my AIC, for blood sugar, cholesterol and others tests on October 5, 2011 and it was 5.6 (normal ranges are 4.8-5.9). Cholesterol was 94 HDL was 33 and LDL was 48. I cannot be happier!

October 25, 2011 was my birthday and I have lived over a half a century. For the past ten years, I have celebrated my birthdays with taking many, many medications. This time, for the first time in over two months, I truly felt the joy of losing fifty-four pounds because, so far, I am not going through the agony of poking my fingers for diabetes blood sugar test, or taking a variety of medications for high cholesterol and high blood pressure. This is truly a great joy!

My life and eating habits have completely changed. I take time to eat (Mindful eating), eat slowly and only eat what I know is good for my body. I do not have indigestion or acid reflux, and I am not taking any of the medications that were previously prescribed to me due to my weight issues. I have learned to take care of my body and so can you!

Weight loss is a total lifestyle transformation to change a bad habit. A bad habit can be replaced by a positive habit. This is what has worked for me. I do not wait until I am too hungry to eat. I have learned to plan to eat every 2-3 hours every day. It takes practice and a lot of patience.

One other thing that has helped me tremendously in reducing my weight is writing down everything that goes into my mouth (This may sound outrageous.) I assess at the end of the day or week to see where I could improve. Another thing that has helped me lose and continue to lose weight is getting in to a routine exercise. This is something that can be done slowly. I got to the gym 5-6 days a week for 45-60 minutes each time. If, for some reason, I cannot go, I do home dance and that has been very helpful.

I started slowly especially after I was out of shape for a while. I started with walking around the block two times a week. I had the music on, but changes were very slow. I argued with myself that the benefits of walking was that I need not drive to the gym. I can dress comfortably and there is no need for competition. The disadvantages of walking are, it can get boring and chances of going back to the house sooner are higher. However, if you live in a location or country where walking or physical work is part of the daily routine, then your focus would be concentrated on what you eat more.

I made up my mind that there must be something I can do to improve my health rather than being scared, settling for less and depending on medication as a short cut.

Kaiser Permanente also offered *"Wellness with Diabetes"* which I attended for four weeks. During one of the classes, the instructor gave basic information about what to do to prevent infection.

I set goals for myself. Food is the main factor for weight gains. Too much eating may be caused stress, anger, lack of emotional and social support especially those who live alone.

My weight gain was a combination of eating wrong foods, medication a lack of regular exercise and being an emotional eater. I have changed my eating habits established a healthy lifestyle for a long life.

Some medications can increase a person's weight. There are many factors combined that can be blamed for weight gain, nevertheless, we all can make a decision on what changes we can do to thrive, live well and longer.

Being overweight can also lead to other delusions or symptoms such as high blood pressure, stroke, diabetes, depression, stomach and intestinal problems, chronic fatigue syndrome, and stress. Death never gives us a warning. I decided to make lifestyle changes for my health. Do not get me wrong, I do know that there are some diseases that are irreversible.

If you have a disease that you can do something about then take action.
weight loss Why wait?

Most people including myself dream of a day of peace and quietness. Many have thought of seeking out counseling and a good trainer to be healthy again. Many long for a time to be off the high blood pressure, high cholesterol and diabetes medications.

Losing weight is a struggle for many people. You need motivation to get started with weight loss. You need determination and support from family members. As you can imagine, the people close to us can help us succeed or fail.

I endured a lot of stress regarding immigration status. My body did not return to a homeostatic state, which resulted in chronic exhaustion and illness. My prolonged stress was waiting for the immigration status to change. The stress was more than fifteen years, which contributed to other diseases in the body.

At one point, I thought I was sabotaging my weight loss for personal gain. This can happen unconsciously, for example, if someone is fearful of a meaningful relationship, the chances of keeping the weight on can be a way of keeping the opposite sex at a distant.

I knew, I could not be my own doctor, but I had to do something otherwise, I was going to an early grave. One of the first things that I did was to break these psychosocial stressors into small parts. I made a list and prioritized what to do first. The first priority was weight loss. Self-esteem was not an issue for me. My cultural frame of reference was that heavier people were wealthier. I also saw a therapist during this time. I changed my eating habits and exercised regularly.

Another element was communicating with friends and family members. They helped me cope with stress. Prayer and meditation are other ways of reducing stress. It has always worked for me.

Today as I write this message, my weight has dropped to 199 pounds. I cannot stress enough what difference this has made in my life. My blood pressure has dropped drastically, I have energy and I feel good. For a long time, my weight never bothered me coming from a culture where "the more weight one has, the richer people think or assume you have". Subsequently, this has changed now.

I hope that by sharing these struggles, hopes and plans will inspire you to make changes in your life. Being overweight has many disadvantages. It can affect your health, your relationship and even the price and comfort of an airplane flight.

This is the first time in so many years that I have felt very good about my health. I feel energized, excited, free and happy to be over a half a century years old.

I hope those reading about my journey of weight loss will make some small changes for their health and life in general. I am also grateful to God's goodness in so many different ways!

I have chosen to write about my problems with weight because I chose to lose the weight, and because I was aware that my medical problems arose from my weight. There are some people who have had other debilitating diseases whose major symptom are weight loss, but chose not to lose weight.

This morning I thought of my life in the past half a century and the families I have worked with and I realize the problems of weight need to be confronted honestly. Some family members will never mention the excess weight because of fear of hurting someone's feelings.

There are no quick fixes for weight loss. If you grew up in a farm, you will understand the law of harvesting. "A farmer reaps what he sows". For any change to be effective, a dieter should plan for a long-term solution. This plan should include good nutritional practices, regular exercise, and open communication with your physician and family members, as well as, relaxation and meditation techniques.

Trying to lose weight is not an easy task! Dieting or changing your eating habits temporarily is easy. For example, if a friend is getting married in a month's time, you are motivated to lose weight your dress will fit. Unfortunately, you may gain everything you lost at the wedding party.

Having a healthy body, healthy mind, and healthy finances is not an easy undertaking. I have experienced a lack of all three. This is not an easy short cut to weight loss. You need to change the way you live your life. You do not have to wait until there is a life threatening experience like mine to change. Remember, you only have ONE LIFE TO LIVE! If you are unconcerned about your weight, you still need a healthy mind and healthy finances.

I think back on the milestones I have passed in my life and I realize that the commencement of positive changes stemmed from some form of bad news.

i) Becoming a born-again Christian in November 1981-after a painful and traumatic divorce
ii) Emigrating to the US as an adult in September 1995-after the death of my 2 brothers
iii) Going back to school at the age of 35 in September 1995 when my ex-husband remarried
iv) Changes in my health and lifestyle in February 2011 when I was diagnosed with diabetes

I have lost seventy pounds (70 pounds) since February 2011. As I write this biography of my journey to America by air and how American food and lifestyle led me to gain over one hundred pounds. I cannot be happier with the progress I have made to change my life and lifestyle in general.

I never thought I would reach this state of mind and body.

I feel great as I write this memoir. I know beyond every reasonable doubt that if I did not make these healthy choices, I would not be here today. I had reached a point in my life where I had given up on many things; including losing weight and feeling normal again.

After losing my only job in 2009, I was desperate and lonely. I felt betrayed and angry within myself. In addition, my house foreclosed in June 2011. I finally moved to a rented place. All these events were too much to take in one year.

Today, things are much different for me. I lost seventy pounds one year between February 2011 to February 2012. I am also no longer taking any medications for high blood pressure, high cholesterol and diabetes.

If there is anything, I would thank God for more than any silver or gold is my good health. I could not be happier!

My goal was/is to lose seventy more pounds within a year or two.

My plan was to start with short-term goals. I would exercise at least three to four times a week. I would eat when I was hungry and I would eat the right foods.

In the past, I had tried several quick ways of losing weight but I quickly regained the weight. This time I got some tips from Kaiser Permanente, and I followed through their suggestions. Today I can see the results.

There are many theories why weight loss does not work for some people. I have realized that there are small daily steps that can lead to permanent weight loss. Important things that I did to change my health were; eating breakfast, containing-protein, carbohydrates and a vitamin. Exercising regularly 4-6 times a week, eating every 2-3 hours and low fat foods, eating more white meat and less red meat, more greens and fruits with less sugar, eating less saturated fat, sleeping 6-8 hours, and avoiding or managing stress in your life. Every little lifestyle change helps to bring you a healthy tomorrow.

As much as obesity is a health problem, achieving weight loss and maintaining that loss is a complex problem. Making small changes, exercising, talking to your physician, family, friends or colleagues and eating low carbohydrate or fat free foods is the key to successful weight loss.

It is a good idea for me to watch myself closely for changes in my health, and to be sure to contact my doctor.

Almost any activity that gets me moving and strengthens my muscles is good for my health and can help move me towards my weight goal. Forty-five minutes of brisk exercise burns 250 to 350 calories. If you have not been exercising regularly, start slowly and gradually increase the duration, the frequency, and exertion you apply to your exercise routine.

No matter how much we want something; all journeys begin with first step. I really wanted to lose weight and improve my health. I started with a first step of attending twelve weeks of classes and another four weeks for diabetes class, both at Kaiser Permanente.

I learned that an old dog could be taught new tricks. It worked for me. I am now enjoying my second half of my century. My grandmother lived to be one hundred and three year (103) old. My wish and prayer is that I will live to be one hundred and five years old and still have my own teeth.

I have shared with others some coping strategies, but did not apply the formula to my own life. Antecedents – TV food commercials did not influence me. Deep within me, I knew they were advertising for money. However, I must admit that Pizza commercials influenced me in some ways. I watched these ads and ordered a pizza.

Consequences – my weight gain was close to three hundred pounds. I developed diabetes, which was my wake-up call. I do not drink alcohol neither do I smoke. I go to the gym 4-5 times a week. I eat every 2-3 hours and small portions. I eat more fruits with less sugar, greens and vegetables, fish, chicken, sweet potatoes, squash, and pumpkin and limit myself to three eggs a week I do eat cheese at least 5 pieces a week. I take my vitamins daily.

CHAPTER 11

Mind Changes, Exercises and Simple Foods

These are good exercises that I have learned to do: gardening, hiking or biking, joining health club classes, doing exercises at home or while doing chores at home like vacuuming. Several health clubs such as LA fitness offer a variety of fitness classes such as spin (recumbent bicycles), Body Works, Pilate's, Yoga, and many others. It is a good idea to find out what is offered, try a few classes and find one you enjoy. I joined Zumba dance class (Latino Heat). Dancing can also be a good way to exercise, which you can do at home or by joining dance classes at the local gyms, schools or dance studios.

In any life situation, balance is the key. I cannot focus on physical exercise alone and neglect the spiritual, mental and social aspects of life.

As I mentioned earlier, being diagnosed with diabetes was my turning point to lose weight.

Attitudes are important. Early attitude theorists proposed that attitudes have three basic components: the cognitive, the affective or emotional, and the behavior or conative. People have differing attitudes about many things. Nevertheless, where does this attitude came from? As you might suspect, there is no single answer to this question. Some attitudes are based on direct experience with the attitude object, whereas others are acquired less directly. Some people have the attitude that no matter how much or little I eat, it will not make any difference in my weight, so why bother?

Attitude and behavior are related. Do attitudes predict behavior? Choosing a healthy diet is something that many people unfortunately struggle with, and I was no exception. The temptation of fast food and other easy choices leads people to pick whatever is available or seems to tastes the best.

There are simple and cheap ways to lose weight. I tried for several years chronic dieting which made it harder to lose weight. What has worked for me is mindful eating. This sounds simple, but it works. Think and prioritize beforehand what you want to eat. What is appealing to the eye might not be good for the stomach. Some people say we first taste food with our eyes. If you have a plate of colored foods, think of the rainbow colors, it suggests that you are including a variety of food groups in your diet, which nutritionally is more inclusive than one color.

There are many different diets out there including low carbohydrate diets and the truth is that most of them will achieve weight loss if they are followed correctly. This does not mean always doing what the diet says every moment of every day. What is more important is how you deal with the inevitable occasion when you eat too much or feast on foods that are not on the plan. If you can write this off and return to the plan without giving yourself a hard time, you are likely to succeed. Everybody has those days. The important thing is to let him or her accepts the temporary set-back and continues with your diet plan

It is also important to find a diet that you can easily follow. Low carbohydrates diets suit many people because the rules are quite simple. As the name suggests, the diet consists of avoiding or limiting foods that are high in carbohydrates. These include bread, pasta, potatoes, rice and other grains. Sugar is also a carbohydrate. Once I understood what these foods were, it was a simple matter of dish choices. You can also find healthier alternatives to the bad carbohydrates and replace them with healthier options. For example, instead of eating white rice or pasta, opt for brown rice or pasta; if you must eat bread, eat only small portions of whole wheat bread or grain breads instead of white bread.

Being on low carbohydrate dieting means the dieter will get most of his or her daily calories from meat, dairy and other high fat products. This can lead to high cholesterol and other problems related to a high intake of saturated fats. Seek medical advice before starting this type of diet or any kind of diet. Sometimes weight loss is good in the early stages but people cannot handle the restrictions in the longer term and start to deviate from the diet. Self-determination and motivation play a big role in permanent weight loss.

One of the problems that many people have with low carb dieting is the elimination of bread and pasta. On this diet, there is no more toast, spaghetti or pizza! Many of the foods that are quickest to prepare are based around carbohydrates. Burgers in their buns, fries, sandwiches, pasta and sauce are all high in carbohydrates. Beer and other alcoholic drinks are high in carbohydrates too. It is true that alcohol is generally restricted on any diet, because it is high in calories and very low in nutritional value.

Still many foods can be enjoyed on a low carb diet. If you are fond of meat, you will delight in the opportunity to consume beef, chicken and other animal products. The popularity of these diets is clear from the length of time that they stay on the bestseller lists. It is just a matter of what suits you. Low carb dieting works for many people.

Whatever state of mind you are, weight loss is not all about food! Everything needs to change including the mind, body and spirit. Good healthy eating begins with a small step and a determination to change.

Many of the foods that I have decided to eat more of have also helped with my weight loss, such as sweet potatoes, squash, pumpkin, eggs (limit 3 per week) fish, beans, and green tea. I take tea with 1% fat milk 2-3 times a day. Any time is teatime as we used to say in Kenya.

Depression is treatable with modern antidepressant medications and short-term psychotherapy.

The cultural pressure for weight loss is mostly on women. Could it be because of what the television and media portrays as the ideal weight? I have come across very few men who talk about their weight or trying to lose weight. For the sake of good health, all people including children need to watch their food intake and do regular exercise.

Sometimes, we fulfill other's expectations of us. For example, a wife who is constantly yelled at, or belittled can feel that she is not good enough. Her response may be to eat uncontrollable using food as a comfort. This may lead to weight gain. Her husband may continue to belittle her because he thinks no one else will have her.

Making choices that are in our best interest should be a priority in our lives. It is important to take care of our spiritual, physical, and mental needs.

Physical fitness is important. You may have been motivated to "get healthy or into shape". There are many benefits to being physically fit. (1) You will look younger, (2) You will live longer, (3) You will feel healthier, (4) You will feel good about yourself and have great positive feeling about yourself.

The mind is a powerful thing! As I began to tell myself that changing my eating habits was a good thing, my perception improved. During my twelve weeks at Kaiser Options, the instructor gave us different menus to try. The menu was designed to reflect one's physical needs bases on one ones' height, weight and age. My menu included 1500 calories a day. I thought to myself, there is no way I can survive on so little food. After several months into the program, I was able to reduce my calories intake.

CHAPTER 12

Summary

During the period I gained most of the weight, there was a lot of stress going on in my life. There seemed to nothing I could do about it. I no longer suffer from stress about immigration status.

However, changing the pattern does not have to be hard. Simply take a few moments to think about it. Our attitude is critical when it comes to choosing the right food. Only I can determine which food is most appealing to me. I realized that I loved bread and peanut butter. Well, I had to change this and, then the journey of weight loss began.

I learned how, when and what to eat, a notion which I thought was ridiculous at the time. I also attended diabetes classes for four weeks and learned all I needed to learn to make changes for my health. I weighed two hundred and seventy nine pounds (279 lbs.).

A few months into the program, my daily intake of calories was 1500. I look back now and I believe in the power of the mind. My mind was telling me that I could not survive, while in reality, I could. As much as I struggled mentally to accept that I could not consume fewer calories per day, I actually did it!

Depression affects different people in different ways. Some people lose interest in food or cannot motivate themselves to shop and cook, so they lose weight. While others find that, they want to eat more and more when they are unhappy and gain weight.

Some medications could also increase weight. Check with your doctor and read the package insert of all medications. My medications increased my weight and depression made me eat more and choose the wrong foods.

Other psychosocial stressors stemming from housing, job, medical, relationships and family are still present in some form. I can handle them by taking care of myself so I can have the strength to face other challenges in my life.

Diabetes scared me to death! I saw myself losing my leg, my eye or other parts of my body. I could not wait for that to happen. This was my turning point! The most significant result of the life changes I made after this scare is that I am off all medications for high blood pressure, high cholesterol and diabetic medications. I no longer check my blood sugar twice a day.

I have mentioned that I am off all my many medications. This may not be automatic for all people who lose weight. I guess, for me there were many side effects from the medications, I had to ask for higher intervention. Again, know your body. Discuss with your doctor and make small changes-slowly! I have asked myself these questions. "Why did I wait this long"? Did I want to die. These two questions made me take a U-turn to change my health life early in 2011. Weight loss is a life long journey and total lifestyle change is essential. One small step is just the beginning.

For any weight loss to be successful, you need patience and the willingness to follow instructions. The five simple steps for permanent weight loss are:

i)   Eating right, choose low carb-balanced meal,
ii) Eat every 2-3 hours
iii) Get regular exercise, 3-6 times a week,
iv) Get enough sleep 6-8
v)   Meditation and prayer
vi) Cultivate a healthy social network.

Well, one week is not enough for permanent weight loss. A more realistic timeline would be two- seven years. I have learned the following: Eat healthy diet; Get plenty of exercise; Get enough sleep 6-10 hours a night; Manage stress in a healthy way; Avoid unsafe activities; Visit the doctor as needed or yearly.

I have learned that, to live a long life, my eating habits and other life choices had to change. The saying '*you cannot teach an old dog new tricks*' does not apply here. Any one of us can make changes to their lifestyle and learn new tricks. I also learned that going over 4-5 hours without food slows metabolism causing the body to burn less fat than normal.

I have made my mistakes and learned to get up and start anew. The most important point in a successful diet is to continue the fight. I have learned from my failures as well as my successes. Do not use a mistake as an excuse for giving up. The only way to achieve my goal permanently was to make a commitment to become a healthier person. I remember that eating normally includes eating more some days and less other days. I have learned to enjoy food in moderation and I have every chance of avoiding these bad diet mistakes.

I was one of those people a year or so ago who did not take care of herself. I changed my lifestyle. If you struggle with weight problems and health related issues, it is not too late to get started today.

Weight loss is a journey that starts with a first step. Sometimes we want a quick fix but not ready to do the work. My question is. "What do I need to conquer in your life"?

Many of us would like a quick fix of almost anything. However, good things in life take time and effort to achieve. It takes time to find a mate, build a career, get a college degree, raise a family, and it takes time to lose weight. None of these things can be done overnight. You need patience, persistence, and commitment. I have succeeded because I started with small steps. I also made it my goal to eat right every 2-3 hours. Eat small portions. Eat fruits with less sugar. Eat more greens, lentils, black beans, spinach, collard greens, chard, and salad with lemon or tiny bit of nonfat dressing.

I am writing from a personal experience, weight loss is not that simple. It is hard work but there is a reward. Simple steps of eating small portions of food are critical.

I had challenges, struggles, discouragement, loneliness, desperation, defeats and despair. I got support and lack of support from friends and family. At the end of the day, it was my life at stake. I decided to do what was necessary to work this time for me. I have only one life to live. I would like to live it well and productive!

Being a mental health therapist did not help me control my moods, hunger or eating habits. I look back now and know the techniques I used to help others struggling with weight loss, relationships and other life's skill.

It is not a good idea not to eat for a long period. This can lead to a drop of blood sugar, which produces more craving and hunger. Not eating regularly can make it harder to control your choices of food at the next meal, snack or the portions. Try to have a healthy snack available at all times. Snacks can include nonfat plain Greek yogurt, 2-4 strawberries, string of cheese, or a100-200 calorie Snack. These will help keep your blood sugar and insulin steady and your energy level high.

I am making wise decisions about reasonable, practical and realistic weight loss goals.

I would strongly encourage you to take steps on managing your weight. Talk to your clinician or physician about how to start making changes in eating and physical activity to improve your weight and overall health. You can learn more about weight loss, healthy eating, and physical activities by emailing me @ HYPERLINK "mailto:wlac.com@gmail.com" wlac.com@gmail.com, or snail mail to Betty Odak, PO Box 10908 San Bernardino, CA 92423, or by phone-562-522-8008. You can also visit HYPERLINK "http://www.comingtoamericabyair1995.com" http://www.comingtoamericabyair1995.com HYPERLINK "http://www.weightlossandculture.com" http://www.weightlossandculture.com

www.ingramcontent.com/pod-product-compliance
Lightning Source LLC
Chambersburg PA
CBHW060218290526
45789CB00003B/1314